© Healthcare Financial Management Association, 1996

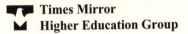 **Times Mirror**
Higher Education Group

Library of Congress Cataloging-in-Publication Data

Zimmerman, David R.
    The healthcare customer service revolution: the growing impact of
managed care on patient satisfaction / David Zimmerman,
Peggy Zimmerman, Charles Lund.
      p.   cm.
    Includes index.
    ISBN 0–7863–0893–1
    1. Patient satisfaction. 2. Medical personnel and patient.
3. Medical care—Quality control. 4. Hospitals—Administration—
—Case studies. I. Zimmerman, Peggy. II. Lund, Charles. III. Title.
R727.3.Z56 1996
362.1'068—dc20   95–43460

Printed in the United States of America
1 2 3 4 5 6 7 8 9 0 BS 2 1 0 9 8 7 6 5

THE HEALTHCARE CUSTOMER SERVICE REVOLUTION

The Growing Impact of Managed Care on Patient Satisfaction

DAVID ZIMMERMAN

PEGGY ZIMMERMAN

CHARLES LUND

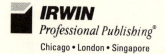
IRWIN
Professional Publishing®
Chicago • London • Singapore

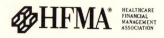
HEALTHCARE
FINANCIAL
MANAGEMENT
ASSOCIATION

THE HEALTHCARE CUSTOMER SERVICE REVOLUTION

The Growing Impact of Managed Care on Patient Satisfaction